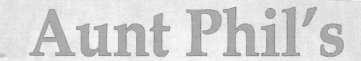

Aunt Phil's

Gratitude

Journal

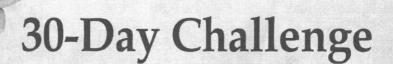

30-Day Challenge

By Laurel Downing Bill

Embrace Gratitude For A Happier Life

Every day we hear about terrible things happening around us. The news often is filled with terrifying stories of violence, hateful political strife and catastrophic world events.

It is not surprising that you might feel like you are constantly surrounded by negativity.

But if you can tune out the television, turn off the phone and not read a newspaper for a day or two, you will realize that you have most of what you need and want in life to make you happy. You have people who love you, food on your table and a warm (or cool), comfortable shelter.

The antidote to a negative attitude is being grateful for what you have right now.

Gratitude can transform you.

I created this 30-day challenge journal as a simple way for you to practice gratitude. Once the challenge is complete, I hope that acknowledging what you are grateful for will become a daily habit that will have a transformative effect on your life.

Happy journaling!

Laurel Downing Bill

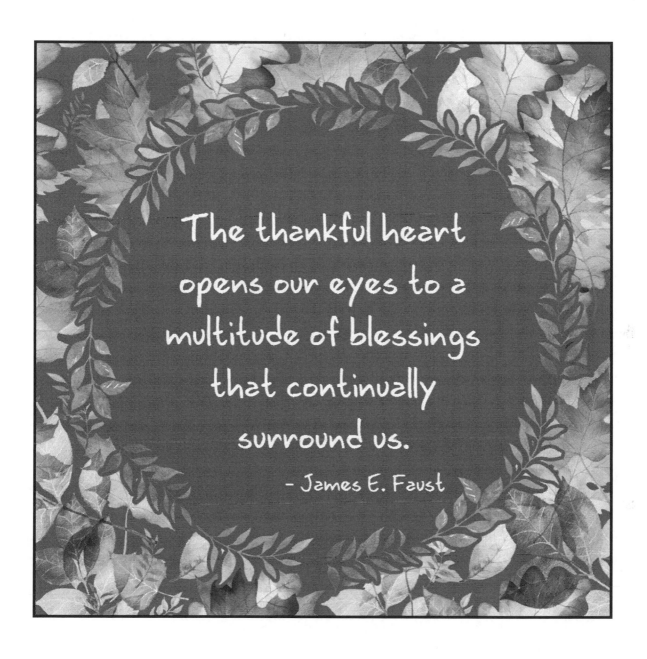

The thankful heart
opens our eyes to a
multitude of blessings
that continually
surround us.

– James E. Faust

Printed in the United States of America
Aunt Phil's Trunk LLC
First Printing November 2019

ISBN: 978-1940479-81-1

Day 1

What is your happiest childhood memory? Describe what happened, who was there and why you think you were so happy then. How can you bring that happiness back into your life now?

_____
_____
_____
_____
_____
_____
_____
_____
_____
_____
_____
_____
_____
_____
_____
_____
_____
_____
_____
_____
_____
_____
_____
_____
_____
_____

Day 2

Who is the one friend you always can rely on? How has this friend helped you recently? How can you show your appreciation for this friend?

_____
_____
_____
_____
_____
_____
_____
_____
_____
_____
_____
_____
_____
_____
_____
_____
_____
_____
_____
_____
_____
_____
_____
_____
_____
_____
_____
_____
_____
_____

Day 3

List 10 hobbies and activities that bring you joy. Why do you find them so enjoyable?

_____
_____
_____
_____
_____
_____
_____
_____
_____
_____
_____
_____
_____
_____
_____
_____
_____
_____
_____
_____
_____
_____
_____
_____
_____

Day 4

Describe a family tradition that you are most grateful for and why.

_____
_____
_____
_____
_____
_____
_____
_____
_____
_____
_____
_____
_____
_____
_____
_____
_____
_____
_____
_____
_____
_____
_____
_____
_____
_____
_____
_____
_____

Day 5

What is one thing you've learned this week that you're thankful for and why?

_____
_____
_____
_____
_____
_____
_____
_____
_____
_____
_____
_____
_____
_____
_____
_____
_____
_____
_____
_____
_____
_____
_____
_____
_____
_____

OFTEN PEOPLE ASK HOW I MANAGE
TO BE HAPPY DESPITE HAVING NO
ARMS AND NO LEGS. THE QUICK
ANSWER IS THAT I HAVE A CHOICE.
I CAN BE ANGRY ABOUT NOT HAVING
LIMBS, OR I CAN BE THANKFUL THAT
I HAVE A PURPOSE. I CHOSE

gratitude.

NICK VUJICIC

Day 6

What is a recent purchase that has added value to your life. How has it added value to your life?

_____

_____

_____

_____

_____

_____

_____

_____

_____

_____

_____

_____

_____

_____

_____

_____

_____

_____

_____

_____

_____

_____

_____

_____

_____

_____

Day 7

What is biggest lesson you learned in childhood? How can you be grateful for that lesson?

_____
_____
_____
_____
_____
_____
_____
_____
_____
_____
_____
_____
_____
_____
_____
_____
_____
_____
_____
_____
_____
_____
_____
_____
_____
_____
_____
_____
_____

Day 8

List 10 ways you can share your gratitude with other people in the next 24 hours.

_____
_____
_____
_____
_____
_____
_____
_____
_____
_____
_____
_____
_____
_____
_____
_____
_____
_____
_____
_____
_____
_____
_____
_____
_____

Day 9

Name and write about someone you've never met, but who has helped your life in some way.

_____

_____

_____

_____

_____

_____

_____

_____

_____

_____

_____

_____

_____

_____

_____

_____

_____

_____

_____

_____

_____

_____

_____

_____

_____

Day 10

How can you pamper yourself in the next 24 hours?

_____

_____

_____

_____

_____

_____

_____

_____

_____

_____

_____

_____

_____

_____

_____

_____

_____

_____

_____

_____

_____

_____

_____

_____

_____

_____

_____

Of all the characteristics needed for both a happy and morally decent life, none surpasses gratitude. Grateful people are happier, and grateful people are more morally decent.

Dennis Prager

Day 11

What is your favorite way to enjoy nature? (i.e. walking in the woods, sitting on the beach, hiking in the mountains, etc.). Why does this activity bring you happiness?

_____
_____
_____
_____
_____
_____
_____
_____
_____
_____
_____
_____
_____
_____
_____
_____
_____
_____
_____
_____
_____
_____
_____
_____
_____
_____

Day 12

How is your life more positive today than it was a year ago?

_____
_____
_____
_____
_____
_____
_____
_____
_____
_____
_____
_____
_____
_____
_____
_____
_____
_____
_____
_____
_____
_____
_____
_____
_____
_____
_____
_____

Day 13

What is your favorite part of your daily routine? Why?

_____
_____
_____
_____
_____
_____
_____
_____
_____
_____
_____
_____
_____
_____
_____
_____
_____
_____
_____
_____
_____
_____
_____
_____
_____

Day 14

Describe what other people like about you.

_____

_____

_____

_____

_____

_____

_____

_____

_____

_____

_____

_____

_____

_____

_____

_____

_____

_____

_____

_____

_____

_____

_____

_____

_____

Day 15

What is your favorite holiday and why do you love it? How can you bring some of that happiness into your everyday life?

_____
_____
_____
_____
_____
_____
_____
_____
_____
_____
_____
_____
_____
_____
_____
_____
_____
_____
_____
_____
_____
_____
_____
_____
_____

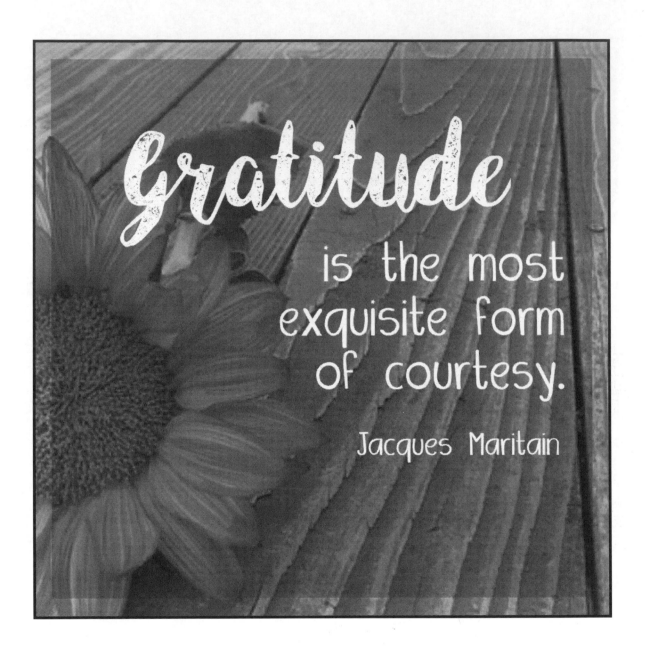

Gratitude is the most exquisite form of courtesy.

Jacques Maritain

Day 16

List 10 skills you have that most people don't possess.

_____
_____
_____
_____
_____
_____
_____
_____
_____
_____
_____
_____
_____
_____
_____
_____
_____
_____
_____
_____
_____
_____
_____
_____
_____
_____
_____
_____

Day 17

What do you love most about your country? Why?

_____

_____

_____

_____

_____

_____

_____

_____

_____

_____

_____

_____

_____

_____

_____

_____

_____

_____

_____

_____

_____

_____

_____

_____

Day 18

If you're single, what is your favorite part about being single? Or if you're married, what is your favorite part about being married? Why?

_____

_____

_____

_____

_____

_____

_____

_____

_____

_____

_____

_____

_____

_____

_____

_____

_____

_____

_____

_____

_____

_____

_____

_____

_____

Day 19

Write about someone who makes your life better.

_____

_____

_____

_____

_____

_____

_____

_____

_____

_____

_____

_____

_____

_____

_____

_____

_____

_____

_____

_____

_____

_____

_____

_____

_____

_____

Day 20

List 10 things you are looking forward to in the next year.

_____

_____

_____

_____

_____

_____

_____

_____

_____

_____

_____

_____

_____

_____

_____

_____

_____

_____

_____

_____

_____

_____

_____

_____

_____

_____

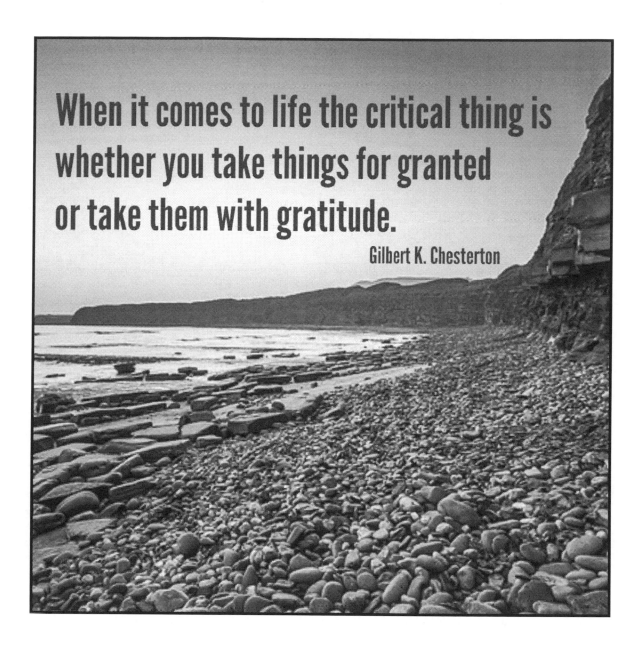

When it comes to life the critical thing is whether you take things for granted or take them with gratitude.

Gilbert K. Chesterton

Day 21

What is today's weather like and what is one positive thing you can say about it?

_____
_____
_____
_____
_____
_____
_____
_____
_____
_____
_____
_____
_____
_____
_____
_____
_____
_____
_____
_____
_____
_____
_____
_____
_____

Day 22

What is one thing about your health for which you are most grateful? Why?

_____

_____

_____

_____

_____

_____

_____

_____

_____

_____

_____

_____

_____

_____

_____

_____

_____

_____

_____

_____

_____

_____

_____

_____

Day 23

Describe a "perfect day" that you recently had and why it was so perfect for you.

_____
_____
_____
_____
_____
_____
_____
_____
_____
_____
_____
_____
_____
_____
_____
_____
_____
_____
_____
_____
_____
_____
_____

Day 24

List 10 things that you take for granted, which might not be available to people in other parts of the world – like indoor plumbing, clean water, etc.

_____
_____
_____
_____
_____
_____
_____
_____
_____
_____
_____
_____
_____
_____
_____
_____
_____
_____
_____
_____
_____
_____
_____
_____

Day 25

What is one thing you look forward to enjoying every day? Why?

_____

_____

_____

_____

_____

_____

_____

_____

_____

_____

_____

_____

_____

_____

_____

_____

_____

_____

_____

_____

_____

_____

_____

_____

_____

_____

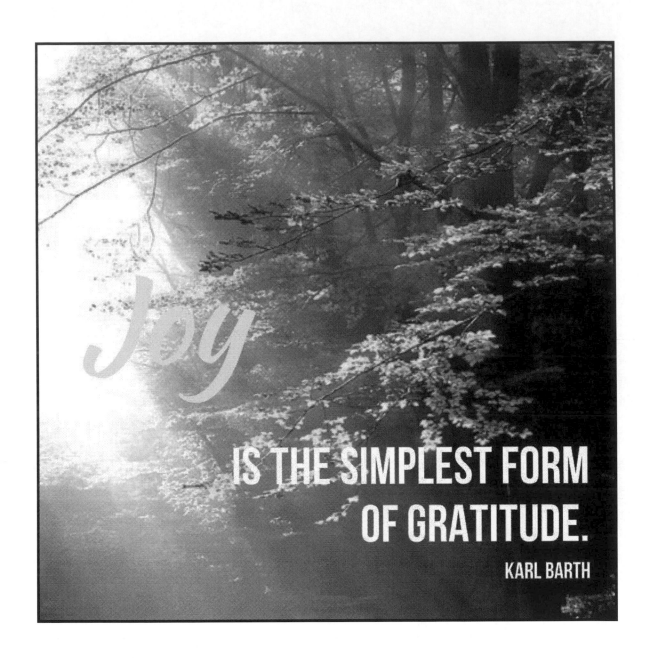

Joy

IS THE SIMPLEST FORM
OF GRATITUDE.

KARL BARTH

Day 26

Describe a recent time when you felt really at peace. Is there any way you can get that feeling again and be grateful?

_____
_____
_____
_____
_____
_____
_____
_____
_____
_____
_____
_____
_____
_____
_____
_____
_____
_____
_____
_____
_____
_____
_____
_____
_____

Day 27

List 10 things you have now that you didn't have five years ago.

_____
_____
_____
_____
_____
_____
_____
_____
_____
_____
_____
_____
_____
_____
_____
_____
_____
_____
_____
_____
_____
_____
_____
_____
_____

Day 28

Describe an experience that was painful, but that made you a stronger person.

_____

_____

_____

_____

_____

_____

_____

_____

_____

_____

_____

_____

_____

_____

_____

_____

_____

_____

_____

_____

_____

_____

_____

_____

_____

_____

_____

Day 29

What do you love most about the current season? Why?

_____
_____
_____
_____
_____
_____
_____
_____
_____
_____
_____
_____
_____
_____
_____
_____
_____
_____
_____
_____
_____
_____
_____
_____
_____
_____

Day 30

Write about someone in your life with whom you frequently disagree. Then describe the qualities you most like about this person.

_____

_____

_____

_____

_____

_____

_____

_____

_____

_____

_____

_____

_____

_____

_____

_____

_____

_____

_____

_____

_____

_____

_____

_____

_____

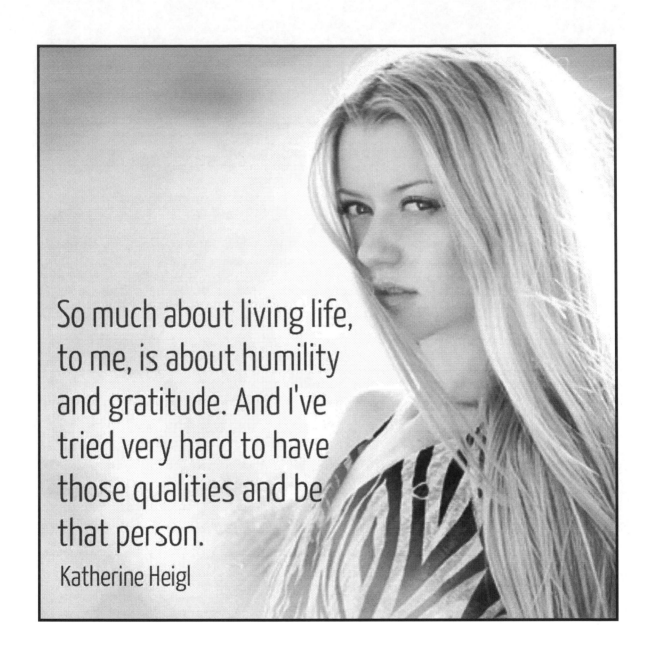

So much about living life, to me, is about humility and gratitude. And I've tried very hard to have those qualities and be that person.
Katherine Heigl

Made in the USA
Middletown, DE
25 April 2022

64702706R00040